Fit. Confident. Unstoppable.

28 DEVOTIONS TO
KICKSTART OR REIGNITE YOUR
FITNESS JOURNEY!

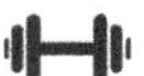

BY JENNA J ALLERSON

A big thank you for the beautiful cover and internal layout design completed by Kristen Kimbrough.

For more information: contact jenna@jennaallerson.com
www.jennaallerson.com

Print ISBN: 979-8-9897410-0-7
eBook ISBN: 979-8-9897410-1-4

To my firstborn, Owen.

This book wouldn't be possible without you. I never would have found my voice and my deep faith in Jesus. I am forever grateful for you, son. I love you today, tomorrow, and always.

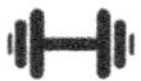

"THE FIRST
STEP TOWARDS
GETTING
somewhere
IS TO DECIDE
YOU'RE NOT
GOING TO STAY
where you are."

-John Pierpont "J.P." Morgan

Table of Contents

Welcome

"Movement is a medicine for creating change in a person's physical, emotional, and mental states."
- Carol Welch

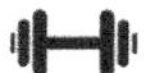

Hello, reader. From now on, I'll be referring to you as a friend. I'm so happy that you've chosen to invest in yourself and your fitness journey.

This book was created with a heart to help you start or restart your fitness journey using encouragement, motivation, and practical advice. My prayer is that you'll be able to sustain your fitness long after you finish these 28 days.

This journey is not only physical, but emotional as well. It's important to reflect. At the end of this book, you'll find space for your why, your goals, and a tracker to log your workouts over the next 28 days. This space is a judgement-free zone for you to explore and to be able to look back years from now and see how far you've come.

Now, let's get started! I hope these next 28 devotionals keep you motivated and encouraged. I am here cheering you on every step of the way. Jesus is cheering for you. **You've got this!**

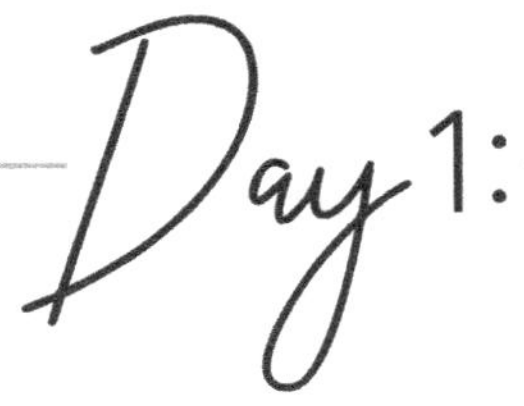

Day 1:

DARE TO START (OR START AGAIN)

*[7]And though your beginning was small,
your latter days will be very great.
Job 8:7 (ESV)*

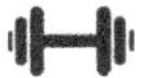

After a significant injury to my foot, I didn't know if I would ever run again. Six months after my injury, I tried to do some slow intervals on the treadmill. It did not go well. My foot and ankle were incredibly sore and swollen afterward. It scared me. I felt less than.

A couple of months later, I was on a trip with my running group in San Antonio, Texas. We had all registered and committed our travel plans from Minnesota to Texas months earlier (when I was still able to run). My plan was to run the half marathon. My reality when I arrived in Texas that December was that I was going to be walking the 5K. I couldn't believe I was going to travel that far to essentially walk 3.1 miles.

But our Lord is so good, and He had other plans for me that December weekend. I walked that 3.1 miles with my close friend Cheryl. We talked about everything—motherhood, marriage, the loss of jobs, all the real stuff you don't see on social media. Soon, the miles were over, and we were at the finish line. I felt new life in me after that walk. I wasn't alone.

The next day—the day of the half marathon—all of us who weren't running the half marathon woke up early to cheer on our friends and eventually meet them at the finish line. While we were encouraging the runners as they ran by, one runner caught my attention. He was an older gentleman who had a significant physical impairment. His legs were uneven. When he ran, it looked like he had on one high heel and one flat. But that didn't stop him. He had so much joy and crossed the finish line with a huge smile.

Soon after, our friends came around the corner. They were about to cross the finish line—some with smiles and some with tears and exhaustion. They wore their emotions on their faces. But they did not stop. Our friend Nancy crossed the finish line, completing the longest race she'd ever run. I was so proud of her. I knew the work that went into getting her to that day. Tears welled up in my eyes.

I knew I needed to begin again—and I did. And so can you! Dare to begin.

Dig Deeper:

Be proud of yourself. Celebrate you for beginning again or starting your journey for the first time!

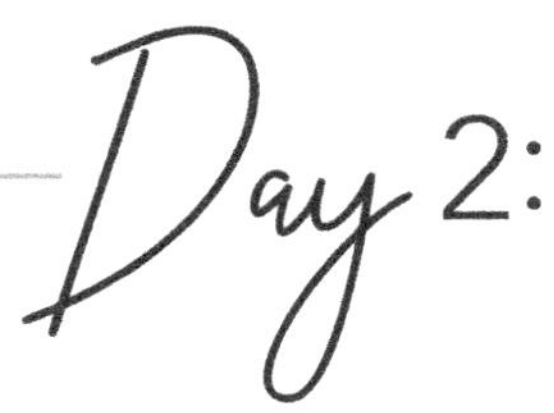

WHAT IS YOUR WHY?

[31]So, whether you eat or drink, or whatever you do, do all to the glory of God.
1 Corinthians 10:31 (ESV)

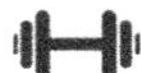

I have pondered this verse a lot. Whenever you set out with a new goal or start a new journey, a mentor will usually ask you why. Why are you setting out to reach this goal? Why are you beginning this journey? Why are you creating a healthy lifestyle?

Finding my why for a healthy lifestyle took me a couple of tries. When I set my why on earthly things such as wanting to lose weight or fitting into a certain dress, the why never seemed to hold. It never kept me disciplined when my motivation was down. It wasn't until I searched deeply that I realized my why is simple.

My why is simply to honor God by moving and taking care of my body. This is a simple why, but it leans into all my other whys.

- I lead a healthy lifestyle to serve my family well.
- I lead a healthy lifestyle so I can serve others well.
- I lead a healthy lifestyle so I can be here on this earth for as long as it takes me to fulfill the purpose God has chosen for me.

Your why is personal to you. You could have a large, overarching why with some mini-whys that lead to your goals. Whatever it looks like for you, choose one that is powerful, one that keeps you going on the days that are hard—the days that are uncomfortable. Those days will happen, but you are stronger than the adversity.

Dig Deeper:

Write down your why in the back of this book today!

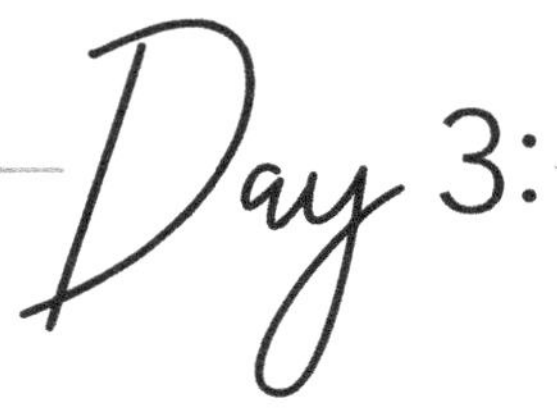

SET A GOAL

[7]But you, take courage! Do not let your hands be weak, for your work shall be rewarded.
2 Chronicles 15:7 (ESV)

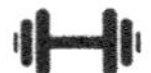

My family is finally at the time when we can all go for a bike ride together. Our sons, Owen and Gus, can ride on their own, and either my husband Matt or I pull the bike trailer behind us with our daughter, Adeline, in tow. It's a great way to get some energy out on long days at home. Fresh air and new scenery are good for the soul.

Just the other day, Matt asked Owen if he wanted to jump on the bikes and go for a ride. It was the perfect fall day. The air was crisp, there was a slight breeze, and the leaves were beginning to change. Owen looked at Matt and asked, "But where are we going?" It seemed like a ridiculous idea to Owen to go on a bike ride without a destination in mind. Matt told him he did have a destination in mind since he needed a couple things at the grocery store. That was enough for Owen. As long as he knew where he was going, he was ready to go.

Much like Owen, we should also know where we're headed when it comes to our fitness journey. If we get up every morning, do the same thing, and have no idea what we're headed toward, it's easy to quickly lose our motivation.

Fitness is a journey. It is not a destination, so you'll need to continually strive toward new goals. That will help keep you motivated and moving forward. I like to choose a fitness program to complete such as the 30 Day Breakaway or the 21 Day Fix. I might set a step goal for the week or month, or sign up for a 5K or 10K and start training. It keeps me going and gives me a goal.

What is your goal? It could be something as simple as completing three workouts a week for four weeks. Once that's completed, you pick something else. Or maybe you want to make it a step goal or sign up for a race. Maybe you set a certain number of minutes per week you want to work out, or maybe your goal is a certain number on the scale.

Whatever it is, make it personal and motivating to you. It won't be easy, but it will be worth it.

Dig Deeper:

Write down your goal. There's space for you in the back of this book. Write it there. Write it on Post-its and put it where you will see it often. Share it with a friend. The more you hear it and see it, the more committed you'll become.

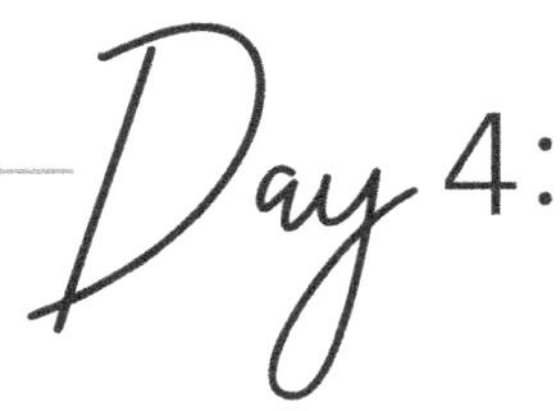

CREATE A PLAN

[4]May he grant you your heart's desire
and fulfill all your plans!
Psalm 20:4 (ESV)

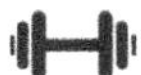

If I'm being totally honest, I must admit that I really don't like to plan. I don't like to have someone tell me when and where I have to be. I like to "feed my flesh" and only do things when I feel like doing them. But there's a problem with that. If we only do things when we feel like doing them, chances are we won't reach the goals we set for ourselves.

That's where a plan comes in. When you have a plan to follow, you don't have to let your mind overthink what you're going to do. You simply do what your plan is for that day—even if you don't feel like it.

I enjoy following the BODi programs. They are virtual workouts I can stream anywhere, and they are all set to a plan ranging in length from 21 to 100 days. I typically choose workouts on a monthly basis. These plans are strategically built to work our entire body in a safe and effective way over a certain amount of time, so I don't have to think about it. I simply just follow the plan.

The Lord wants to give us the desires of our hearts. I know you desire to incorporate fitness into your lifestyle because you are right here with me reading this devotional. Reflect on today's verse, "May he grant you your heart's desire and fulfill all your plans" (Ps. 20:4 ESV). Follow your plan (whatever it is), and watch the Lord fulfill your heart's desires in ways you may not even be able to imagine.

Dig Deeper:

Don't let finding a plan be your hurdle. There are so many plans online now that you can simply google "free (insert your specific workout here) plans," and I promise you there will be a number of choices! Have fun with it!

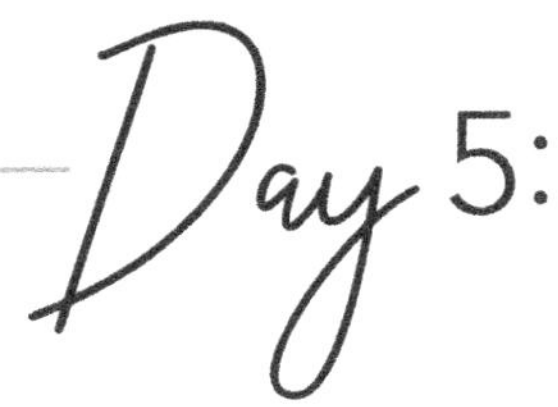

Day 5:

HONOR YOUR TEMPLE

[19]Or do you not know that your body is
a temple of the Holy Spirit within you,
whom you have from God? You are not
your own, [20]for you were bought with
a price. So glorify God in your body.
1 Corinthians 6:19–20 (ESV)

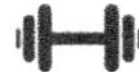

What does it look like to you when you're told to honor God with your body? What does honor look like? According to dictionary.com, honor means "to worship, glorify, or serve (a deity)." God made us in His perfect image. He knew exactly what He was doing. So if we are made to move our bodies, why do so many of us skip it?

We can come up with lots of reasons. Many are simply excuses. Think about it. Do any of our reasons hold up to the ultimate sacrifice Jesus made for us? When we're about say no to our workout, what if we pause and reflect on the ultimate sacrifice Jesus made and say yes instead? Say yes to yourself. And say yes to glorifying Jesus.

The way you honor your body for God is specific to you. He knows everything about you and knows what you need. Take your time, be still, and see where Jesus leads you when it comes to your movement. Is he telling you today to slow down? Is he telling you to challenge yourself?

After my ankle injury, I knew my movement and my way of glorifying and honoring my temple were going to look different. I felt convicted to slow down—way down. Jesus showed me ways to do that. I was still honoring my temple and ultimately honoring Him as well. He was preparing me for something more and knew I needed rest and restoration.

I spent that season stretching, meditating, and practicing yoga. I showed up in a place of silence and spent time honoring my body, which ultimately glorified God. Now I sit here sharing this with you, bringing light to His masterpiece. Without that season of slowing down, I don't think it would have been possible.

Today, if you find yourself lacking motivation or discipline to lean into your fitness routine, do it for the One who made the ultimate sacrifice for us all. Get quiet. Listen to that small nudge in your spirit that's telling you how to move your body today. Honor your temple as an act of gratitude to the One who sacrificed it all.

Dig Deeper:

Go for a walk in nature today. Let your mind take in all the beauty, and immerse yourself in God's creation and the wonder of movement He has given us.

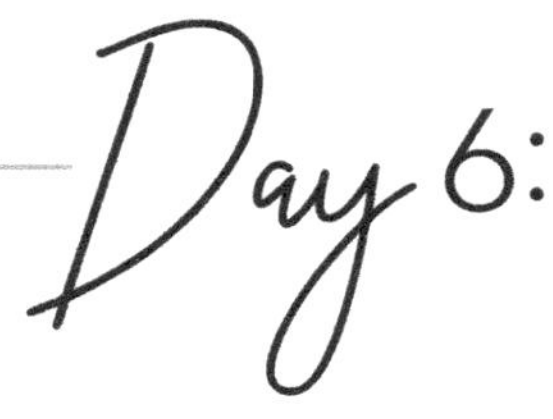

WHAT IF I FAIL?

[16]For the righteous falls seven times and rises again, but the wicked stumble in times of calamity.
Proverbs 24:16 (ESV)

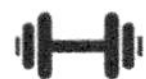

I have a tenacious two-year-old daughter—Adeline Joy. She's determined to keep up with her brothers, regardless of how many times she must try. Before she was two years old, she knew that in order to keep up with her brothers who were six and eight years old at the time, she would need to learn how to perfect her scootering skills.

Let me paint a picture of her. Adeline is in the fourth percentile for height and weight for her age range. She is small but mighty. She could barely reach the scooter's handlebars, but again, that did not deter her. She would jump on that scooter and move her legs until she either found herself crying on the sidewalk or in the grass because she had fallen off.

Did that stop her? Did she beat herself up because she had failed to perfect her scootering skills immediately? No. I don't know the age where we learn about what failure means, but I'm grateful that word isn't in Adeline's vocabulary. After about a week of falling and getting up again, she had her scootering down. She became a little mascot in the neighborhood and was famous for how well she scootered.

Do you know why? She didn't give up!

The same is true for you! There will be days when you're feeling like you are failing at this new fitness journey. Maybe you skipped a workout. Perhaps you're not seeing the gains you want to see. But guess what? You cannot and will not fail if you do not give up on yourself.

Dig Deeper:

Be righteous. Even if you fall down more than seven times, rise again. You will see your victory. You will reach your goals. You cannot fail, especially with God on your side.

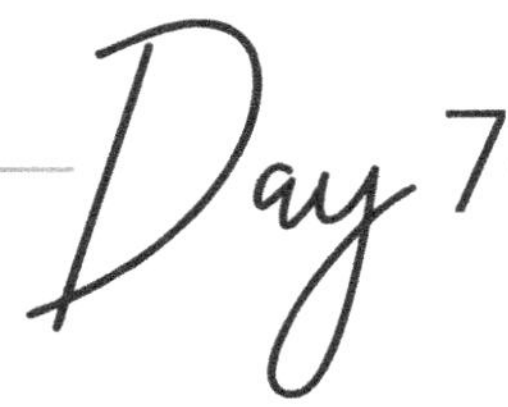

REST IS CRITICAL TO YOUR SUCCESS

[23]Six days you shall work, but on the seventh day you shall rest. In plowing time and in harvest you shall rest.
Exodus 34:21 (ESV)

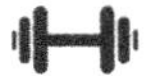

I know how important rest is, but I had to learn it the hard way. I was about nine months postpartum with my third baby (third C-section) and training for a half marathon. At the time, I owned a fitness business and felt I had to do this. My ego had taken over, and my body had to endure the pain.

I began increasing my mileage each week, and soon I was up to a minimum of 15 miles per week (with little sleep being up with an infant overnight). I would do two or three short runs of four-ish miles and one long run a week. My long run was up to eight miles when I had to stop.

At the peak of my training, I was running across a field and stepped in a hole. I heard a crack and knew I was done. I had a level-two sprain and avulsion fractures in my right foot. Looking back now, I can see that I was overworking my joints, giving them limited recovery, and overall not taking care of my body. Yes, a hole in the ground didn't help the problem, but I had done something similar in the past and was able to walk away with minor problems.

This major sprain made me stop dead in my tracks. It made me cancel all my plans. No more training. No more races. It was time to rest. And you know what? It was the first time I had felt peace in months. I knew Jesus was with me, and He was urging me to stop—to rest, to take care of my body.

He sees the whole picture and knows what we need more than we do. A few months after that injury, I went to see an energetic healer for the first time. Without telling her anything about my situation, she told me that if I hadn't been injured, I would have suffered something much worse. God had interceded on my behalf, and I'm forever grateful.

But please do yourself a favor. Check in with your body. Are you feeling fatigued? Exhausted? Anxious? Not motivated? Then give yourself a break. Rest. Recover. And begin again tomorrow or the next day.

Dig Deeper:

Plan a rest day each week—one that works into your schedule. Honor the day as you honor your workout days.

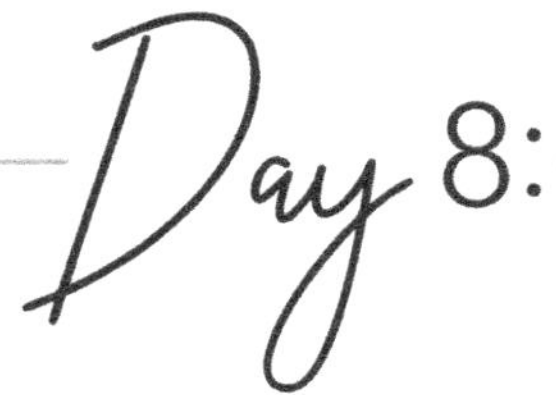

Day 8:

DON'T BE AFRAID TO TRY SOMETHING NEW

[10]Fear not, for I am with you;
be not dismayed, for I am
your God; I will strengthen you,
I will help you, I will uphold you
with my righteous right hand.
Isaiah 41:10 (ESV)

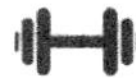

The beautiful way God created us is that we can move our bodies in so many ways. We can swim, dance, lift weights, ride bikes, do yoga, and the list goes on and on. When we're starting something new or beginning something again, it may be easiest to do what we've always done. But most likely part of your picking up this book is that what you've done in the past didn't work or didn't work long term.

I've been consistent with my fitness for most of my adult life. In my 20s, all I knew was to go to the local fitness center, work on some machines, and maybe try lifting a few weights. It was my safe zone. I could blend in. I didn't have to be on display in a fitness class. I never had to push myself more than I wanted. It was easy. The problem with easy is that I wasn't getting the results I wanted. I was in the same place I was at the beginning.

After having my children, I had to step out of my comfort zone and try something new. It wasn't feasible for me to take the time or money to invest in a gym membership. I tried many things that definitely pushed me out of my comfort zone, but it made me better. It helped me love fitness even more. It helped me find my "people"—my community. But I was still scared to try new things like a running group or a group fitness class. I found that I wasn't the only one who was scared. The other participants shared that they were nervous too. I wasn't alone.

The greatest news is that you are never alone. Jesus is always with us to give us strength, peace, and confidence as we walk into new situations. Lean into His presence and take comfort. He has you!

Dig Deeper:

Conduct research on new ways you can move your body—ways to help you achieve your set goals. Be bold, and try something new!

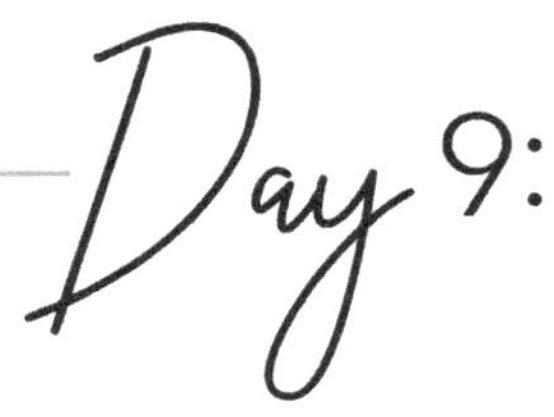

MAKE A DATE WITH YOURSELF

[15]Look carefully then how you walk, not as unwise but as wise, [16]making the best use of the time, because the days are evil.
Ephesians 5:15–16 (ESV)

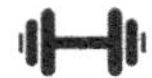

The older I get, the more I realize just how important our time is. It's something we will never get back. So I have to ask you. Are you intentional with your time, or are you reactionary with your time? Does someone else set your schedule, or do you set your schedule?

When I first became a mom, I let time be my excuse for not getting things done, especially things I didn't want to do. Unfortunately, my workout would fall into that category from time to time. I knew it was important for me to invest in my body, but my flesh didn't always want to rise up to the challenge.

The farther I got away from investing time into my body, the more my body suffered. From the outside, others wouldn't have noticed my body suffering. But on the inside, I was a total wreck. My anxiety was through the roof. I never felt at peace or at ease. I knew I needed to make time to take care of myself physically, but it was easier for me to make excuses—until it wasn't.

One morning I woke up drowning in my anxiety—drowning in thoughts of worry, pain, and sadness. I couldn't escape my thoughts. I was miserable. But God (in a way only He can do) led me to Pinterest to a running program. For the first time, something sparked. I felt the smallest twinge of excitement and knew I needed to put on my tennis shoes and go outside for a run.

I laced up my shoes, got my running clothes on, and walked out the door. I began running, and soon I was huffing and puffing. I was out of breath. My legs were burning. I had sweat dripping down my back, my forehead, and even my legs. I was uncomfortable, but you know what? It was the first time I was able to get out of my head and into my body. Running (or any physical movement) became non-negotiable for me. It's my self-care, which ultimately leads to my being able to care well for others.

Now I know that I have to be intentional about my time. Since that first run, I have had two more children. Life doesn't slow down, but I make time for what's important. For me, that looks like getting up 45 minutes before I need to be in the shower so I can get my workout in. I schedule it into my day!

I encourage you to do the same. Make an appointment with yourself, and keep it. The more you honor yourself and remain faithful to you, the sooner it will become a habit.

Dig Deeper:

Tomorrow, set your alarm for 15 minutes earlier. Take a walk outside for 10 minutes! Repeat as many times as you'd like!

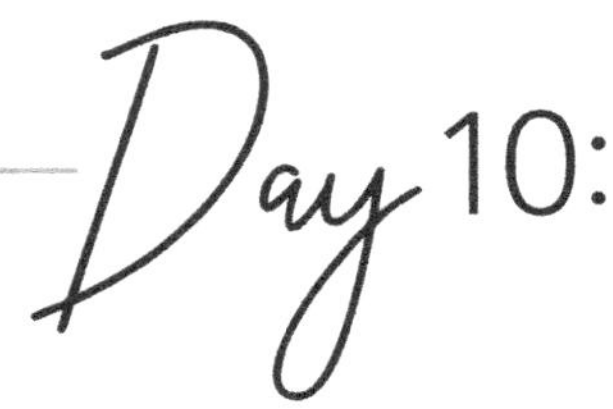

Day 10:

FIND A COMMUNITY

[9]Two are better than one, because they
have a good reward for their toil.
[10]For if they fall, one will lift up his fellow.
But woe to him who is alone when he
falls and has not another to lift him up!
Ecclesiastes 4: 9–10 (ESV)

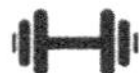

When you are committed to your fitness, you are on a journey. There truly is never an end point. Our bodies are something we need to pour into everyday. The truth is that some days, we're not going to want to pour into them. We're not going to want to make that deposit. We're going to want to sit alone and binge something on TV.

That's where community comes in. It's built-in support. It's built-in accountability. I'm pretty sure it's built-in fun. I'm in the season of life where my schedule is at the mercy of three small children.

About 12 months after giving birth to my third child, I experienced the most significant injury of my life. I was hosting a Mother's Day 5K and kids run at a local park. The kids run was in full swing, and I was sprinting across the field to cheer on my son and help a few runners who had gotten distracted. But I didn't make it to the other side of the course. Instead, I stepped directly into a hole and fell to the ground.

I heard some sort of a snap. I tried to get up and fell right back down. There was no walking on that ankle. Immediately, my community was by my side, lifting me up and helping me to a nearby bench. Within seconds, my ankle was elevated and iced, and I had a dose of ibuprofen. Tears were streaming down my face, and I could see tears in other people's eyes as well. I was in so much pain, but I was surrounded by a lot of love.

That injury took me out of my running game for over nine months. Slowly, I made my way back and planned my "redemption" run with the same community that picked me up months before. They were cheering me on at the finish line, tears streaming down my face again, but this time for a different reason.

I know I'm blessed to have this local community. But if you can't find a local community, I encourage you to find a virtual one. There are many free Facebook groups, Garmin groups, or paid groups such as BODi and Peloton where people will keep cheering you on and looking for you to show up. And who knows? You just might help someone else show up or make their day by cheering them on.

Dig Deeper:

Make an effort today to find a local community. Do a simple Google search, and see what comes up.

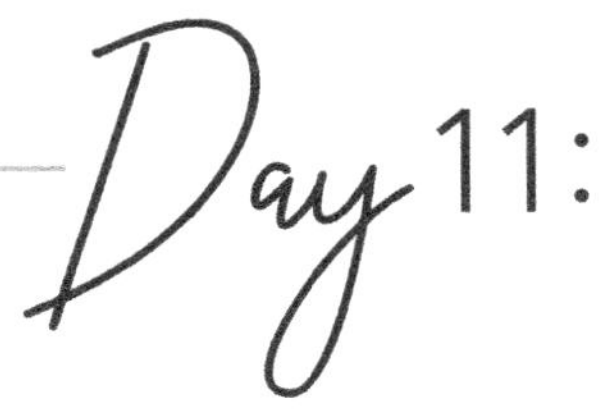

Day 11:

RUN YOUR OWN RACE

[12]Not that we dare to classify or compare ourselves with some of those who are commending themselves. But when they measure themselves by one another and compare themselves with one another, they are without understanding.
2 Corinthians 10:12 (ESV)

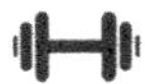

Comparing ourselves to others begins at a very young age. Even before social media seeps in, we begin looking around to see what everyone else is doing. My son Owen has a superpower. Yep, I'm going to call it a superpower (I know, #mombrag). Since a very young age, Owen has been able to run very fast. He even has the reputation of being fast at school (and he's only in third grade). Other mamas are always telling me that's what their kiddos tell them about Owen.

So naturally, we want to support and lean into developing Owen's superpower. Every spring, Owen goes out for track and gives it his all when he runs his races, but there's one thing that seems to always slow him down. He'll be in his lane, close to the finish line, and then he begins to look around. He wants to see where his competitors are. Are they close? Does he need to go faster? And then he slows down because he's so worried about everyone else.

I remind him afterward (after a win or loss) that this is his race and no one else's. I tell him that it doesn't matter what anyone else is doing as long as he's doing his best. And I need to hear that just as much as he does. God has our journey perfectly laid out for us, and if we concentrate on fulfilling God's purpose, we will always end up where we're supposed to be in life and on our fitness journey.

What's your superpower? Is it consistency? Is it strength? Is it a positive attitude? Lean into your superpower today. You have one too. How can you apply it to your fitness journey today?

Dig Deeper:

Reflect on and journal what your superpower is. Own it. Be proud of it.

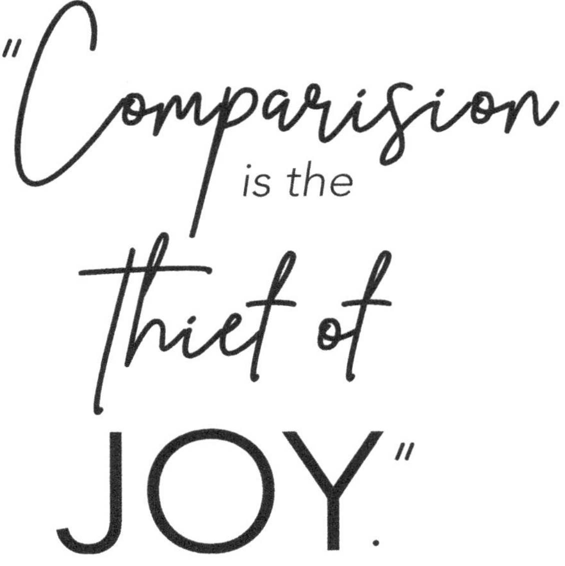

-Theodore Roosevelt

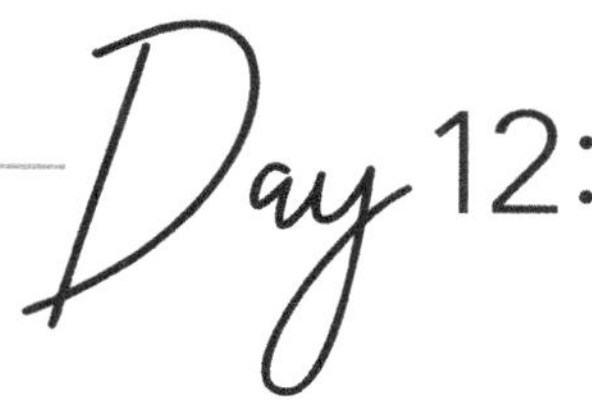

Day 12:

BE BRAVE

[11]Do not be slothful in zeal, be fervent in spirit, serve the Lord. [12]Rejoice in hope, be patient in tribulation, be constant in prayer. [13]Contribute to the needs of the saints and seek to show hospitality.
Romans 12:11–13 (ESV)

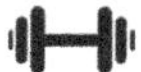

I was at a women's summit last fall, and there was an overall theme to all the speaker's talks—fear. Fear robs us of so many good things in life. We let ourselves get bombarded with all the "what-ifs" about a certain situation—especially a new one. But those what-ifs that we ruminate on aren't the good what-ifs but all the bad what-ifs. In the case of our fitness journey, it could look like What if I fail? What if I don't reach my goal? What if I injure myself somehow? What if I embarrass myself in class? The list goes on and on. (Side note: Do you know that our brain is naturally programmed to go to the negative? We have to intentionally tell it to think positive thoughts.)

The one thing that stayed with me months after leaving the halls of that women's summit is something that Author Rebecca Heiss said. I'll paraphrase it. We always weigh all the risks of what

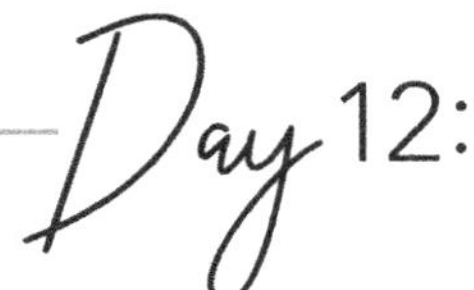

could happen if we do something, but what if we start weighing the risks of something we don't do because we're afraid?

Wow! Mic drop! Just think of that. We never consider what the risks are to the missed opportunities we don't take or the missed rewards we don't reap because we're afraid to start. I want to encourage you to not let the fear of your fitness journey keep you from starting and, more importantly, from continuing.

Be brave, my friend. Reap the benefits for taking the steps into your fitness journey. You've got this.

Dig Deeper:

Are there areas in your life where you're holding back because you're afraid? Lean in, and take a small step forward today—even in the midst of the fear.

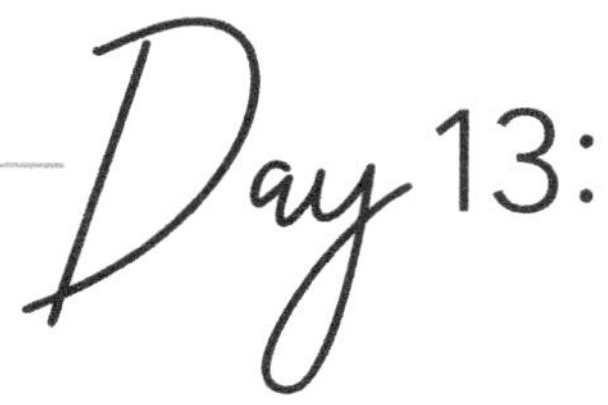

Day 13:

BE KIND TO YOURSELF

*[2]May grace and peace be multiplied
to you in the knowledge of God
and of Jesus our Lord.
2 Peter 1:2 (ESV)*

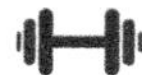

One thing (of course there are many more) I'm guilty of on a daily basis is talking negatively toward myself. It's so easy for me to scold myself when it comes to a missed workout, a missed deadline, or a not-so-good food choice. Instead of showing myself grace and being kind to myself, I immediately go the other route.

The good news is that at least I have identified the behavior, so then I can start working on my inner dialogue. It takes intention every day to rewire my brain to show myself the love I would show to others.

Because you're reading this book, I know you have taken the first step. You have identified that you are seeking a fitness journey. And I know that when starting something new, something uncomfortable, something we may wish we'd started a long time ago, we can be hard on ourselves.

We can critique ourselves if we feel we can't do all the exercises

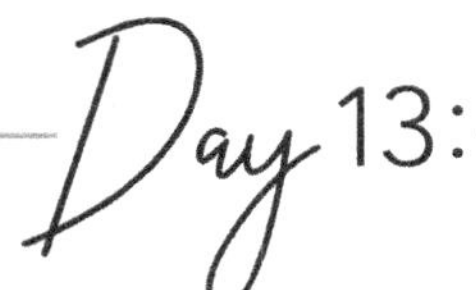

the trainer says or if we can't last as long in the workout as we wish we could. Maybe we begin shaming ourselves for how long it took us to finally take this first step. Maybe we are scolding ourselves for how we look in the mirror. And the thoughts just keep repeating themselves. Unfortunately, that's normal. You must work to change your thinking. Work to change your thoughts. Scolding ourselves isn't going to get us to our goals any faster, but kindness just might.

My prayer for you is that you will be your biggest cheerleader. I will be cheering you on from afar, but I pray that when I can't be there to encourage you, you will encourage yourself. Celebrate the wins, and even when you have missteps on your journey, be kind to yourself. Treat yourself like you would treat your child, your pet, or another loved one with gentleness and love.

Show yourself grace as God shows us grace every day.

Dig Deeper:

How can you celebrate you today?

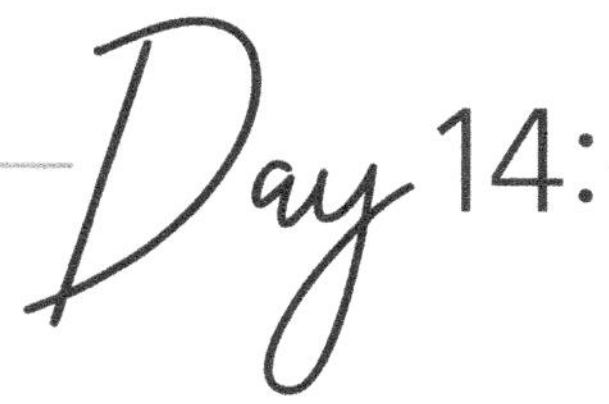

Day 14:

REST, REPLENISH, AND RESTORE

[2]And on the seventh day God finished his work that he had done, and he rested on the seventh day from all his work that he had done.
Genesis 2:2 (ESV)

God can do anything! His powers are endless. He created everything. Knowing that God has the choice to do whatever He wants, I find our verse for today very powerful. God chose to rest on the seventh day. He chose to make the seventh day holy for us. He knew we would need it and set an example for us.

When you're on a fitness journey, you need rest, too, my friend. When we're chasing lofty goals or want to see results happen faster, it's hard for us to stop since we may feel like we're losing momentum. We might feel like we're losing an opportunity to make gains, but we can't look at it like that.

God knows our body better than we do. He created us and knows what we need not only to survive but also to truly thrive. Yes, pushing ourselves to get stronger and healthier is part of that, but so is rest.

Day 14:

According to ACE Fitness, "A day of rest allows your body to repair tissues damaged from the mechanical stresses of exercise. Specifically, rest allows time for the fibroblasts—individual cells that repair damaged tissues such as muscle proteins—to do their job and repair any tissues that need it."

Isn't God wonderful? Resting serves us. It serves so many wonderful purposes, but look how it is specifically and scientifically proven to serve us on our fitness journey. Our rest days allow our bodies to recover so they can come back stronger during our next workout. Have I convinced you yet? I hope so!

Dig Deeper:

Today stretch, meditate, or simply relax. Let your body rest and replenish so it's ready for tomorrow's workout.

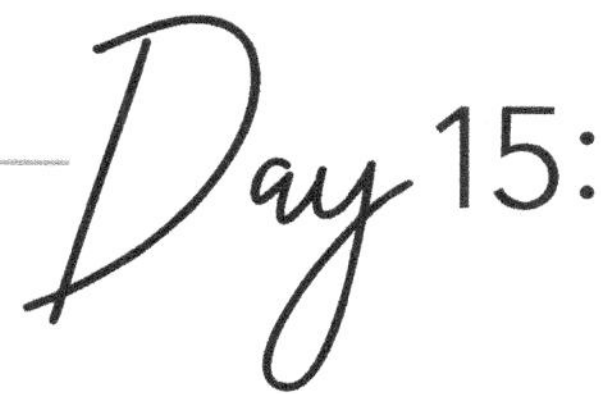

Day 15:

MOVE YOUR BODY WITH GRATITUDE

[16]Rejoice always, [17]pray without ceasing, [18]give thanks in all circumstances; for this is the will of God in Christ Jesus for you.
1 Thessalonians 5:16–18 (ESV)

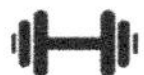

When I was younger, I took everything for granted. I took for granted that my body could move without pain and that I could see, hear, and talk. I could learn, grow, and work. All those things felt like a given—until it wasn't.

Since I turned 30, there have been multiple times when the "given" of moving my body in the way I wanted was taken away from me. While I was pregnant, I needed to change the way I moved. I had to adjust after my three C-sections, my burst appendix, and finally my level-two sprained ankle. I love how God used these experiences to not only humble me but also to teach me how to be grateful for all my blessings.

Now, when I step on the treadmill, my heart is filled with gratitude since I couldn't do this the year before. Because you chose to read this book, it tells me you're able to move your body in some way. I encourage you to fill your heart with gratitude the next time you start your workout. However you're moving, even if you're not at the level you're hoping for, be grateful.

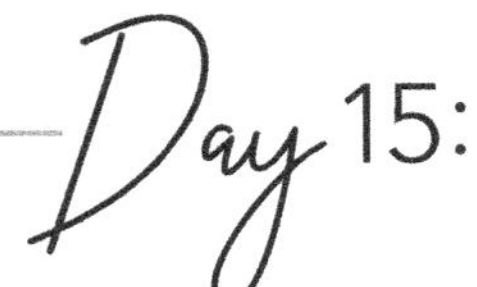

Day 15:

Practicing gratitude is scientifically proven to help us experience less physical pain and discomfort. A study by the University of California, Davis, found that people who regularly practice gratitude experience fewer aches and pains and generally feel healthier than others.

But the greatest gift of practicing gratitude during our workout is that we are able to deepen our relationship with God. When we praise Him for His good work and gifts, we grow closer to Him. What an amazing gift!

Dig Deeper:

Prior to starting your workout, pause and praise God for your body and what you're able to do.

"Develop an attitude of *gratitude*, and *give thanks* for everything that happens to you, knowing that every *step forward* is a step toward achieving something *bigger and better*

- Brian Tracy

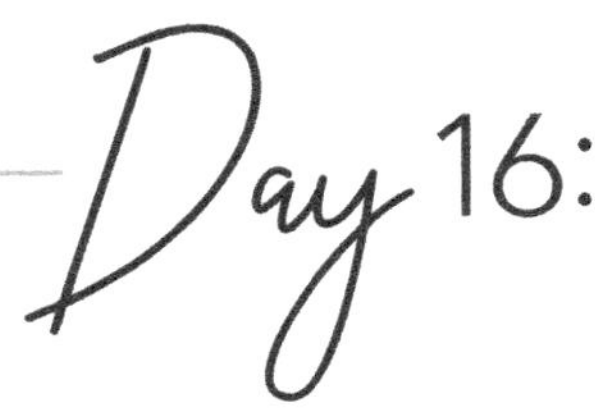

Day 16:

WHAT IF PEOPLE JUDGE ME?

*[10]For am I now seeking the approval of man,
or of God? Or am I trying to please man?
If I were still trying to please man,
I would not be a servant of Christ.
Galatians 1:10 (ESV)*

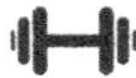

After my second baby, I knew there were certain things I needed to do to ensure that I supported my mental health. I needed to get in movement, and I needed to get out of my house from time to time. With my oldest child, I was confined to my home because he was at high risk for illness, and the isolation sent me into a tailspin.

So when August came along, I was grateful that my son was healthy and born during the summer so I could get outside and walk. I knew I was taking care of myself, but others looked at me through different eyes.

I would get "the looks"—you know, the ones where people's faces say it all. Other times I would get these comments: What are you doing walking already? Shouldn't you be resting? You don't have to rush it; the baby weight will come off. The comments kept coming, but I had to choose to ignore them and know I was doing the right thing for me, my baby, and my family.

Now that I'm far enough outside my postpartum period, I hear other things like this: I don't know how you run those miles. I don't know how you work out so early when you have three kids. I just don't get it.

It's taken me a long time to realize that all these comments are less about me and more about the person saying them. It's easy for me to intellectually rationalize this, but emotionally the comments can start to take a toll. When our emotions take over, we need to lean in and realize that we have our own why and that we are ultimately not trying to gain human approval but rather God's approval, just like today's scripture says.

God's approval reigns supreme over all, and if we keep our eyes on Him, these other comments can begin to feel very small.

When we're on a journey that may be different from those around us, the comments are bound to come. I know this from my own experience and from helping many other women in my fitness business and personal coaching. I just want to encourage you that as long as your heart is yearning to please God and to ultimately honor the temple He has given you, you are on exactly the right path you should follow.

Dig Deeper:

Are you more concerned with what people think or what God thinks about you? Be honest with yourself. If you don't like the answer, what steps can you take to change it?

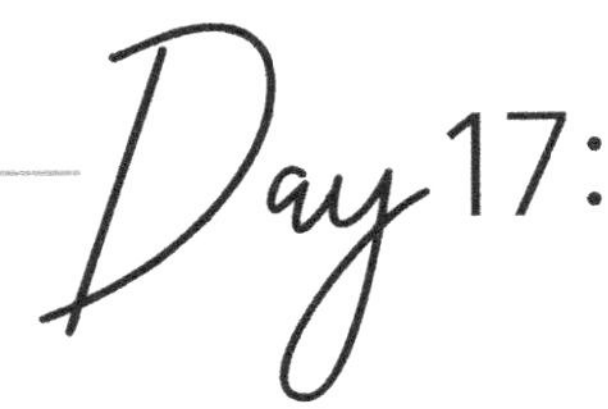

NOURISH YOUR BODY

[29]And God said, "Behold, I have given you every plant yielding seed that is on the face of all the earth, and every tree with seed in its fruit. You shall have them for food."
Genesis 1:29 (ESV)

In order to move our body well, we need to nourish our body well.

When my children were very young, they began to learn about healthy food in preschool, but they were getting confused quickly. There are so many options out there and so many messages that I don't blame them for thinking that it's confusing. It can be confusing for us adults too.

So I tried to simplify it for my children. They would ask me about a specific food, and I would ask them, "Did God create it?" They knew that God created all fruits, vegetables, animals, fish, nuts, and grain. They understood that. If the answer was no or, even worse, they didn't know what it was made of, chances were good that what they were asking about wasn't the healthiest option.

I also added a follow-up question. Does it look like it did when God created it? For example, if they were eating fruit snacks, they would say, "Yes, God created fruit." But I would say, "Does it look like the strawberry on the vine?" And the answer would be no. That helped them realize that even though it may appear healthy, it may not be as healthy an option as the actual strawberry.

And just because they knew it wasn't the healthiest option for them didn't mean they didn't eat it. My kiddos, like many kids, love crackers, fruit snacks, cookies, and more. But for a split second, they at least think about what they are putting in their bodies. I hope that will stay with them as they move into adulthood.

I challenge you today to be really honest with yourself. Are you putting nourishing foods into your body? Are you eating the foods God has provided for us? Is the food in the form God created it, or is it overly processed?

Dig Deeper:

Audit what you're eating, and make small changes, if necessary. God created us perfectly in His image, and He knows exactly what we need.

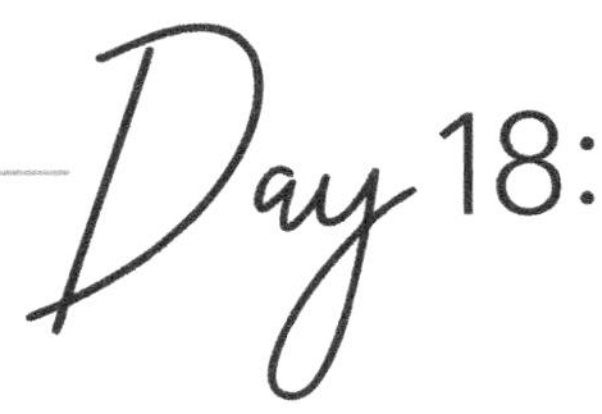

Day 18:

SHARE: YOU ARE INSPIRING OTHERS

24And let us consider how to stir up
one another to love and good works,
25not neglecting to meet together, as is
the habit of some, but encouraging
one another, and all the more as
you see the Day drawing near.
Hebrews 10:24–25 (ESV)

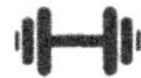

We're so blessed to live in a time when connection is at our fingertips. With a tap on a screen we can check out someone's photos from the other side of the world or even across the street. A lot of time social media gets a bad rap because it can cause more harm than good, but I do believe we can use it as another platform to spread God's love and inspire others.

I grew up on a secluded street just south of the Twin Cities in Minnesota. Our home was tucked away, so it got little traffic. The neighborhood kids played together outside in the streets or on their front yards, so all the kids knew each other's names.

Two doors down from me lived a family of six: two boys and two girls all around my age. I never quite connected with them during our time on that small little street, but the magic of Facebook stepped in almost three decades later and changed my life and fitness trajectory.

My neighbor Chrissi began to share her fitness journey online. Chrissi shows up every day on social media and shares a workout, a fitness tip, or a helpful nutrition hack. If she says she's going to show up, she will. And guess what? She reaps the rewards. She is healthy, happy, and motivated.

I had been watching from afar on Facebook, not saying much but becoming inspired. Eventually, I opened my mind and heart, and we began a fitness journey together. She coached me for many months through my injury and a low mindset and brought me back to my love of running. If she hadn't been sharing, my life would have never changed.

I share this because she had no idea of the impact she was having on my life. And you won't know who you might inspire, ultimately changing their life. It doesn't have to be social media. Maybe it's simply sharing your journey with a friend at work, at the school pickup line, or at church.

Dig Deeper:

Share with someone today. Be brave. Step out. You never know what could happen.

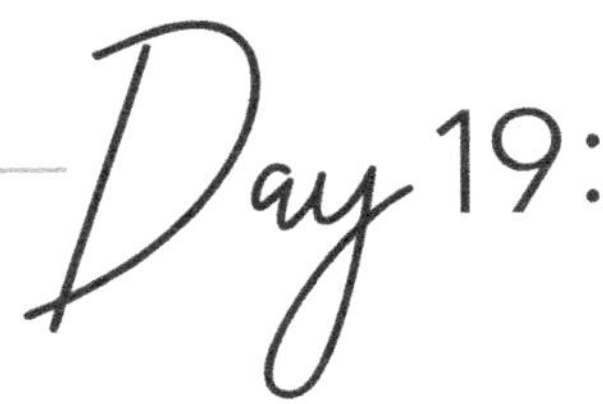

Day 19:

GUARD YOUR MIND

[8]Finally, brothers, whatever is true, whatever is honorable, whatever is just, whatever is pure, whatever is lovely, whatever is commendable, if there is any excellence, if there is anything worthy of praise, think about these things.
Philippians 4:8 (ESV)

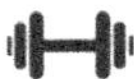

Do you check in with your thoughts—I mean really check in with your thoughts? According to the National Science Foundation, "an average person has about 12,000 to 60,000 thoughts per day. Of those, 80 percent are negative and 95 percent are repetitive thoughts."

When we're starting something new like a new fitness program or beginning again, we need to make sure we're in the right mindset in order to truly succeed. If we're filling our minds with thoughts that tell us we can't do it, we're going to fail before we begin.

So what can we do about it if we're already predisposed to think negatively?

When I was walking through my postpartum anxiety journey after my first child was born, I experienced negative thoughts about 95 percent of the time. I had a hard time concentrating on anything else. I was in a constant state of despair. Our thoughts, after all, are very powerful.

I knew that if I wanted to change the way I was thinking, I would have to be intentional about it. Below are some tools I used to create a more positive mindset, and I hope they will be helpful for you too!

- When I felt my mind starting to wander into the negative, I replaced it with my favorite scripture, Proverbs 3:5–6 (ESV), which says. "Trust in the Lord with all your heart, and do not lean on your own understanding. In all your ways acknowledge him, and he will make straight your paths." I would repeat it over and over until my mind felt at peace.

- I played uplifting songs that made me happy and lifted me up—songs about overcoming and joy! What songs bring you joy?

- I put sticky notes in my car, on my bathroom mirror, and in my planner that reminded me of my strength and the truth of what God says of me.

- I intentionally watched what I was "consuming," and I don't mean what was on my plate. I removed the news, negative TV shows, negative radio, negative podcasts, and more. There's so much media bombarding us every day. Choose wisely what you let into your mind and heart.

Day 19:

Having a positive mindset will not only help you create your new healthy lifestyle when it comes to fitness but may help you see all aspects of your life—your relationship with yourself and others, your confidence, your overall outlook on life—turn for the better.

Dig Deeper:

Check in today. Is it time to make a mindset shift?

"THE HARD PART ISN'T GETTING YOUR *body* IN SHAPE. THE HARD PART IS GETTING YOUR *mind* IN SHAPE."

-Unknown

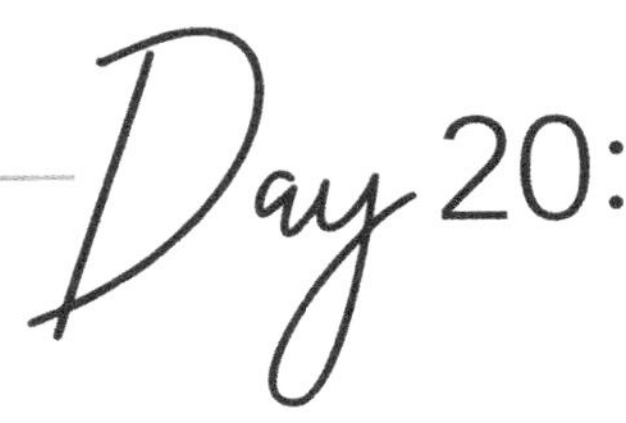

Day 20:

FIND AN ACCOUNTABILITY PARTNER

[17]Iron sharpens iron,
and one man sharpens another.
Proverbs 27:17 (ESV)

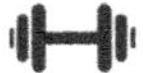

Do you ever find yourself thinking it would be easier to do something by yourself? Then you don't have to involve anyone else's opinions, advice, or timeline. I have fallen into that trap more than once. It's hard for me to put myself out there, admit that I need help, and feel vulnerable with someone. But God created us to be in relationships with others. He created us to be in relationships to make each other stronger and better. And here's the best part. He knows who we need and puts the right people in our lives exactly when we need them.

The proof is in the numbers. An article in *Entrepreneur* stated, "The American Society of Training and Development found that people are 65 percent likely to meet a goal after committing to another person. Their chances of success increase to 95 percent when they build in ongoing meetings with their partners to check in on their progress."

When I began this challenge of writing *Fit. Confident. Unstoppable.*, I knew I would need someone to keep me on track. I love to write, but life gets busy, and it's easy to push aside something that may seem nonessential, even though it brings us joy. As a mom, I'm the first one to push aside my nonessentials to serve my family, and I had a good feeling this passion project would be the first thing to go.

So I enlisted someone special to me, someone God knew I would need to keep going. She has always been my biggest cheerleader, and I trusted that she would see me through to the end. That someone is my Aunt Shar. Every time I finished an entry, I sent it to her. I was always excited to hear what she had to say. She helped bring me to the finish line and I am forever grateful.

Dig Deeper:

Look around for your Aunt Shar. Look around for your biggest cheerleader. I promise they'll want to see you reach your goals and go along with you on this fitness journey.

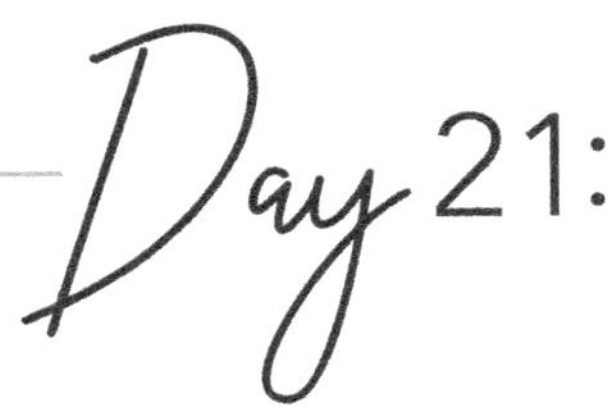

Day 21:

RECEIVE THE GIFT OF SLEEP

[2]It is in vain that you rise up early and go late to rest, eating the bread of anxious toil; for he gives to his beloved sleep.
Psalm 127:2 (ESV)

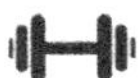

Can I tell you a secret? I'm an achiever. Some may say I'm an overachiever. On every personality test I've taken, achieving consistently comes up as one of my first strengths. On the Enneagram, it's a category all its own. I thrive on achieving, succeeding, and doing, but guess what the problem with that is. All the achieving, doing, and succeeding can leave me feeling exhausted, tired, and empty.

After my third baby, I owned two fitness businesses. We were still in the midst of COVID-19, and there was so much to do. I wanted to do everything I could to make these businesses successful, and I would sacrifice anything—usually my sleep. Every Tuesday morning I woke at 5:15 a.m. to lead a virtual barre class. It didn't matter if the baby was up all night and I was low on sleep, I was there, hoping that if I poured every ounce of me into these businesses, they would succeed—I would succeed. But guess what. They didn't.

On paper, they looked successful. But even though the bank account wasn't empty, I was. God convicted me to stop and reprioritize. What was the first thing I canceled? That early morning class.

Accept God's gift, and prioritize your sleep and rest. When you're starting a new fitness journey or maybe elevating your journey, your body needs extra rest to restore. Remember, rest and sleep are all part of your fitness plan. Rest well, my friends. You deserve it.

Dig Deeper:

Reflect on your sleep. Are you getting enough? Do you need to make changes to start prioritizing better rest?

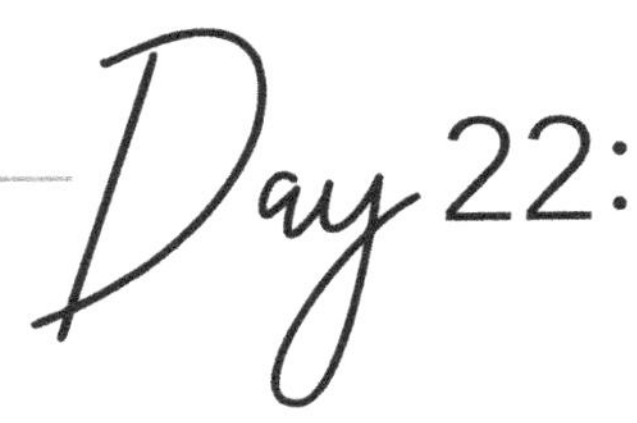

IF IT WAS EASY, EVERYONE WOULD DO IT

13 Enter by the narrow gate. For the gate is wide and the way is easy that leads to destruction, and those who enter by it are many. 14 For the gate is narrow and the way is hard that leads to life, and those who find it are few.
Matthew 7:13–14 (ESV)

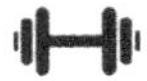

After my oldest son was born, I suffered from extreme postpartum depression. I wanted to take a pill and make all my problems go away, but that doesn't lead to true freedom. I had to put in the work. Did I take a magic pill that helped? Absolutely! But it was just one tool in the toolbox. I had to lean in and put in the work. I had to move my body (even though it was uncomfortable), I had to eat the right foods (even though I wanted junk food), and I had to confront emotions and situations I had buried for years because they held too much pain.

But all the work ultimately led to my freedom. It ultimately led me to you. Without going through that painful and difficult journey, I wouldn't have found my voice. I wouldn't be writing this book, and I wouldn't be the woman I am today.

The same idea is true in our verse today. You are among the few who are walking through the narrow gate, the one that is hard but the one that is ultimately leading you to life. How amazing is that? You are holding yourself to a higher standard, and I'm so proud of you!

We are on day 22 of this fitness journey, and you may be feeling the excitement wearing off. Your motivation may be waning, but I want to remind you that if this was easy, everyone would be doing it. Not everyone is. You are. Be proud. Keep going. You've got this!

Dig Deeper:

Reflect on other places in your life where you've shown up and been among the few. Celebrate you!

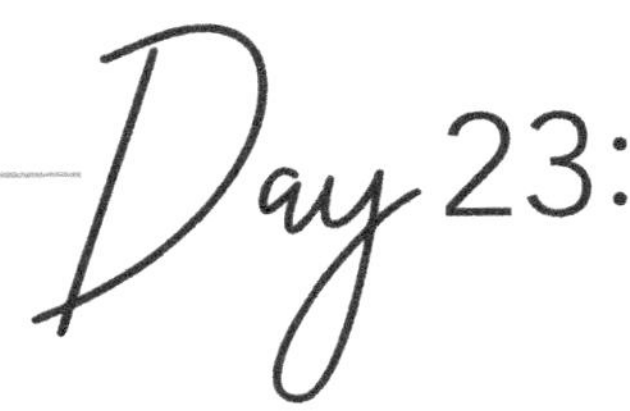

Day 23:

CONSISTENCY IS KEY

[9] And let us not grow weary of doing good, for in due season we will reap, if we do not give up. [10] So then, as we have opportunity, let us do good to everyone, and especially to those who are of the household of faith.
Galatians 6:9–10 (ESV)

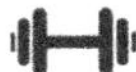

I was at the first grade orientation meeting with my kiddo's teacher for the first time. We were going over all the "stuff" that was going to make our child successful in first grade. There was all the usual stuff—send them with this, read that, reach out with any issues, and on and on.

But the one thing that stuck out to me more than anything was the illustration about making reading a consistent act at home. The illustration showed that after a year of reading only 30 minutes one time a week, a child reads 1,560 minutes. Two times a week at 20 minutes adds up to 2,080 minutes. But if you read only 15 minutes a day five times a week, after a year the child racks up 3,900 minutes! Think about the gains that can happen to a child's literacy after 3,900 minutes of reading.

The same thing is true for you and your fitness. Consistency is key! It will cement the habit and create discipline, even when there's no motivation. The results are in the numbers. You're going to gain so much more when you commit (even a shorter time) most days of the week versus sporadically jumping in and out.

Make a commitment today that you're going to show up. You're going to show up consistently. And you're going to reap the rewards.

Dig Deeper:

What will you commit to? Be realistic. What can you insert it into your current routine? Write it down, and keep the commitment you make to yourself.

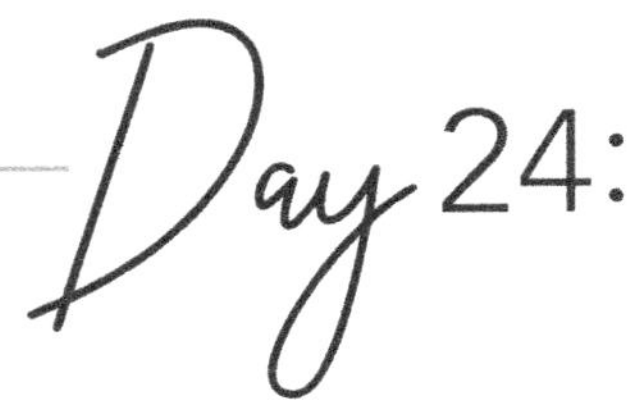

Day 24:

PATIENCE IS A VIRTUE

[12]Rejoice in hope,
be patient in tribulation,
be constant in prayer.
Romans 12:12 (ESV)

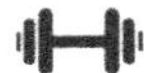

Do you remember those sayings our parents always said when we were younger? You know, the ones that annoyed us. Well, for me, my mother always said, "Patience is a virtue." At the time I didn't really understand what she meant, but I honestly think I need to hear it more as an adult than I did as a child.

Patience has many definitions according to dictionary.com, but the ones that resonated most with me are: "an ability or willingness to suppress restlessness or annoyance when confronted with delay" and "steady perseverance; even-tempered care; diligence."

I don't know about you, but there's rarely a day when I'm not delayed or having to persevere when my emotions get the best of me. Let's be honest. Being patient is hard.

Every single day I pray for patience. I specifically pray for patience when it comes to parenting my children. There's constant fighting, constant noise, and constant delays. I get frustrated.

I lose my temper and I honestly don't like the version of me that comes out sometimes. Sometimes I just want to give up. I want to leave my house and not deal with being a mom for a while, but that wouldn't meet my long-term goal of being a patient, present, and loving mama!

The same goes for our fitness journey. Sometimes we're going to want to give up and throw in the towel. We're going to get tired of putting in the hard work without seeing the results fast enough. We want to see the scale go down. We want to see the weights that we're lifting increase. We want to see our miles become faster. I know this because I want it too. But what I have learned is that we must be patient with our body. It takes time to change. But, if we remain faithful, patient, and consistent we will reap the rewards of our hard work.

God has never promised a life without hard work and tribulation, but His word teaches us to be patient in tribulation. To rejoice in hope and to be constant in prayer. We will reap the goodness of our efforts. It's only a matter of time.

Dig Deeper:

Reflect. Are you a patient person? Are there areas in your life or people in your life you wish you could be more patient with? What's one way you can practice patience today?

"All great ACHIEVEMENTS require time."

-Maya Angelou

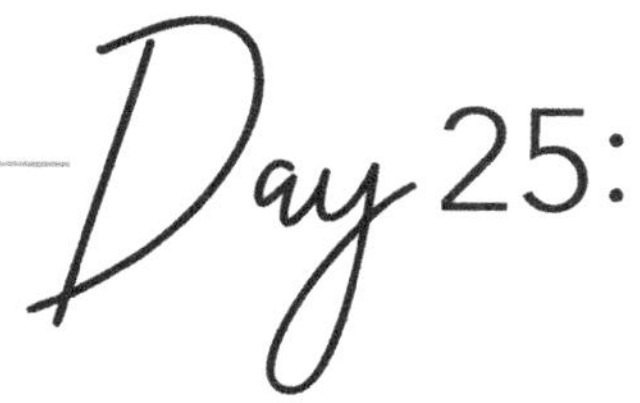

Day 25:

DISCIPLINE OVER MOTIVATION

[7]For God gave us a spirit not of fear but of power and love and self-control.
2 Timothy 1:7 (ESV)

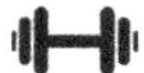

Our Lord is so amazing, isn't He? He knows exactly what we need to truly thrive in life. We see in the book of Second Timothy that the Spirit that lives in all of us makes us courageous—not timid. We have the power, love, and self-discipline to accomplish our goals.

I typically work out in the morning. Even on the weekends, I set my alarm before everyone else's so I can pour into myself before serving others all day long. Do I always have the motivation to get out of my cozy bed while the rest of my family is tucked into their warm beds and sleeping?

The simple answer is no, and that's when discipline kicks in. That's when the love I have for myself kicks in and gets me out of bed to complete that workout for the day. I have to love myself enough to discipline myself.

I think about this a lot when I'm disciplining my kids. Discipline is one of my least favorite things about parenting. I want to be a "fun" mom. I don't want to constantly be redirecting or

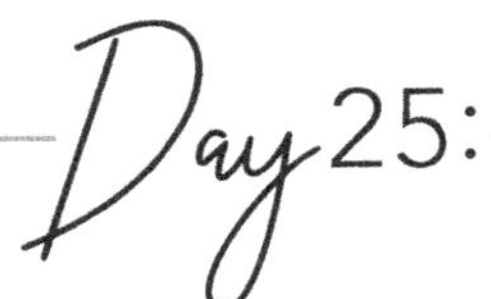

scolding my kids, but then I think of the goals and dreams I have for my children—dreams for them to be kind, generous, and smart (plus a thousand other things). That means sometimes I must discipline them for their own good. I must discipline them because I love them more than I dislike being uncomfortable.

Your self-discipline works the same way. Sometimes you must discipline yourself because your motivation will wane, and it may wane quickly for some. Choose to love yourself. Choose to discipline yourself today. What does that look like for you?

Dig Deeper:

How can you show self-discipline today? Is it your fitness journey? Is it in your eating habits? Is it in what you're watching on TV?

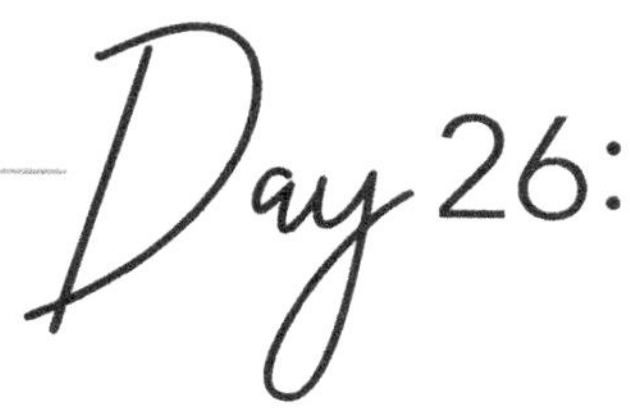

FIND JOY IN THE JOURNEY

[22]A joyful heart is good medicine,
but a crushed spirit dries up the bones.
Proverbs 17:22 (ESV)

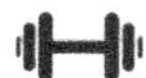

The Lord wants us to enjoy our time here on earth. He doesn't want us to be living with sadness in our hearts and in our bones.

We should do everything with an intention to please God. If God wants us to live joyfully, how can we take our fitness journey and turn it into joy?

Find something you like to do. There is no right or wrong way when it comes to moving your body. Maybe you love to dance. Join a local community education class. Enroll at a dance studio. Maybe you love to be outdoors and take on adventure. Begin hiking at your local parks, or go trail running.

Maybe you prefer slow and intentional movement that also pairs with your mindset. Try yoga, deep breathing, pilates, or barre. Are finances a concern? There are many free options now on YouTube. Just search for what you want and begin moving your body within minutes.

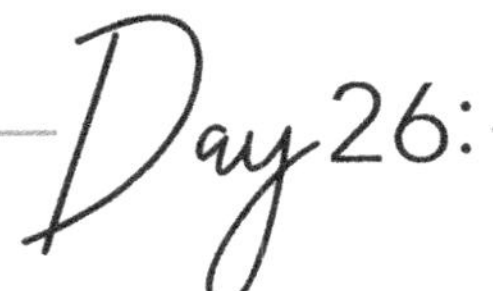

Here's another way to find joy in movement. Find a buddy! Invite a friend on a walk, hike, or run. Talk, laugh, and enjoy each other's company. Doing something with another person helps us stay distracted from the discomfort that may come with physical activity.

Joy may come to you while exercising, even if you didn't intend it. We are so wonderfully made that God rewards us by releasing endorphins into our bodies as we exercise. Endorphin comes from the words endogenous, which means within the body, and morphine, an opiate pain reliever. Put together, that means endorphins are natural pain relievers. They are feel-good chemicals because they can make you feel better and put you in a positive state of mind (see www.clevelandclinic.org).

Now go and crush that workout, and feel all the joy from that endorphin release!

Dig Deeper:

Reflect on what, when, and where you find joy during your workouts.

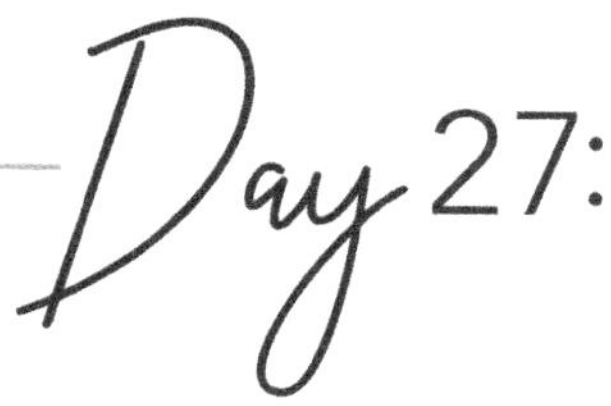

Day 27:

DO NOT GIVE UP

[13]I believe that I shall look upon the goodness of the Lord in the land of the living! [14]Wait for the Lord; be strong, and let your heart take courage; wait for the Lord!
Psalm 27:13–14 (ESV)

Before I had my third baby, I was in the best shape of my life. I had completed my first half marathon. I had just run my fastest 10K. I could see definition in all the right places, and the scale was nearing the pre-baby mark from my first baby. It wasn't unusual for me to meet my running group, complete seven miles, and still be able to do more.

In addition, I had just purchased a local fitness franchise and was teaching multiple strength classes a week. I felt on top of my fitness and nutrition game. But something was missing. I looked at my two boys and envisioned a little one next to them. I knew this was the time—the time to have another baby. I prayed about it. I spoke to my husband, and within a month, our baby was on the way.

I stayed active my entire pregnancy. I ran until I was 28 weeks along. I followed the doctor's orders, but I kept moving.

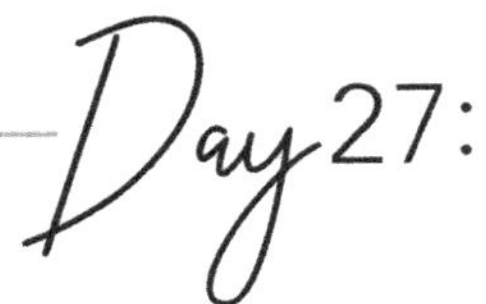

Day 27:

After all, I had to keep up with two little boys and my business. Everyone kept telling me I would bounce right back after I had the baby. But guess what. I didn't.

I gained almost 45 pounds with my pregnancy. The first 30 pounds were relatively easy to shed. But after two years, I still find myself in the battle to shed those last 10 to 15 pounds. I'm doing the right things. I'm exercising. I'm eating well. I'm limiting my sugar and alcohol. I know what to do, but why am I not seeing what I want to see?

Sometimes God is working on what's best for us versus what we want. I went to my annual physical two years after having Adeline, and to my delight, my cholesterol was down 61 points and my blood pressure was down 20 points, putting me in the healthy range for both.

God revealed to me that the efforts are working even when we may not see the results we are looking for. He's always working for our good. I know the external results will come if I just keep showing up.

Do not give up on you. Do not give up on your journey, for you, too, will reap a harvest soon. You will see the results you're searching for if you do not give up!

Dig Deeper:

Reflect on gains you're experiencing off the scale! Non-scale victories are just as important as the ones on the scale.

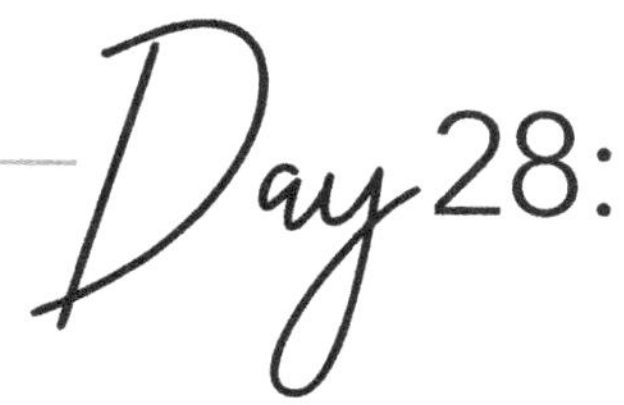

Day 28:

CELEBRATE! YOU DID IT!

[23]"And bring the fattened calf and kill it,
and let us eat and celebrate. [24]For this
my son was dead, and is alive again;
he was lost, and is found."
And they began to celebrate.
Luke 15:23–24 (ESV)

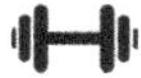

Congratulations, my friend! You did it!

You made it through your 28-day journey. I hope you're feeling Fit. Confident. and Unstoppable. Completing a 28-day program is not easy to do. It takes discipline, motivation, tenacity, and heart to keep going. You have all these things and more. This is just the beginning for you. As I always say, fitness is a journey, not a destination.

I absolutely love our scripture verses for celebrating your accomplishment today. Just like the father in this scripture thought his son was dead, you may have thought your ability to create habit and become physically active was also dead. But it's not! You are at the end of this first chapter on your journey and ready to embark on the next one.

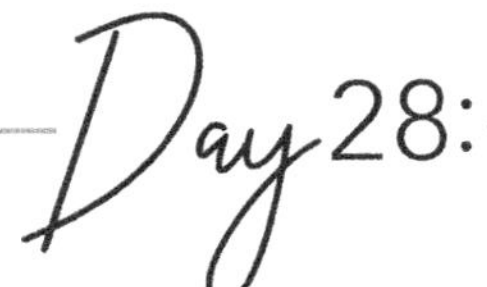

Day 28:

Now celebrate yourself—whatever that looks like for you. Maybe you're treating yourself to a special massage, a treat, or a new outfit. Whatever it is, do it with joy in your heart, knowing that you just finished something hard. You did that, my friend.

After you celebrate and recognize your accomplishments, make sure to set your next goal. You are not done! You're only just beginning.

Congratulations, my friend! I'm so proud of you.

Dig Deeper:

Celebrate you today! You did it. How can you treat yourself? After you celebrate, decide how you're going to keep going! Remember, you're on a journey.

Thank You!

Jesus, thank you for leading my steps to this exact moment. Lord, thank you for equipping me for everything that I needed to complete this dream.

To my sweet husband, Matt. Thank you for supporting me through every journey and adventure that I bring to you. Life with you is by far my favorite adventure.

To my children. You teach me more every day than I could teach you. Thank you for making me the woman that I am today. So much of it is because of the three of you. I love you all so much.

To the amazing community of women that I get to run with and do life with. You are forever imprinted in my heart, and I am forever grateful for your love, support, and humor.

To my family, especially my Mom, Dad, and Aunt Shar, thank you for always believing in me. Thank you for encouraging me to keep writing. Thank you for loving me.

To all of my readers, my new friends. Thank you for coming along with me on this 28-day journey. I pray that it blesses you and that this is just the first chapter in your fitness journey.

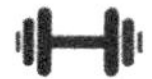

Your Why

Your Goals

28 Day Fitness Tracker

Monday Exercises:

Tuesday Exercises:

Wednesday Exercises:

Thursday Exercises:

Friday Exercises:

Week: Month:

Saturday Exercises:

Weekly Goals:

- [ ] ______________________
- [ ] ______________________
- [ ] ______________________
- [ ] ______________________
- [ ] ______________________

My Motivation:

Sunday Exercises:

Notes / Reminder:

28 Day Fitness Tracker

Monday Exercises:

Tuesday Exercises:

Wednesday Exercises:

Thursday Exercises:

Friday Exercises:

Week: Month:

Saturday Exercises:

Weekly Goals:

- [ ] ____________________
- [ ] ____________________
- [ ] ____________________
- [ ] ____________________
- [ ] ____________________

My Motivation:

Sunday Exercises:

Notes / Reminder:

28 Day Fitness Tracker

Monday Exercises:

Tuesday Exercises:

Wednesday Exercises:

Thursday Exercises:

Friday Exercises:

Week: Month:

Saturday Exercises:

Weekly Goals:

- [ ] ______________________________
- [ ] ______________________________
- [ ] ______________________________
- [ ] ______________________________
- [ ] ______________________________

My Motivation:

Sunday Exercises:

Notes / Reminder:

28 Day Fitness Tracker

Monday Exercises:

Tuesday Exercises:

Wednesday Exercises:

Thursday Exercises:

Friday Exercises:

Week: Month:

Saturday Exercises:

Sunday Exercises:

Weekly Goals:

- [ ] ____________________
- [ ] ____________________
- [ ] ____________________
- [ ] ____________________
- [ ] ____________________

My Motivation:

Notes / Reminder:

Notes

Notes

Notes

Notes

Made in the USA
Monee, IL
21 March 2024

54843498R10049